FOR SABRINA,

I LOVE YOU.

I LOVE YOUR SOUL.

LIVE WELL
BE WELL
LOVE WELL.

Conscious Living Through Cancer
Discover a Lifetime of Wellness Beyond the Illness

To contact the author, visit
www.good4me.ca

ISBN 978-0-9947254-0-0
Printed in Canada

# CONSCIOUS LIVING THROUGH CANCER

## Discover a Lifetime of Wellness Beyond the Illness

By Linda Morinello

# CONTENTS

## DEDICATION

*This book is dedicated to everyone who is walking along the cancer path. May your travels be transformative and inspiring.*

# Preface

I had never considered myself a professional writer or author, and yet I realize that I have been writing this book in my head for many years. When I was diagnosed with lymphoma I knew that I had a message to share. I realized that my destiny was to share it with others to help them in their cancer journey.

When I started to map out what the book could be I realized that it was many things. I wanted to offer a book that contained ideas, thoughts, a little humour, and questions to reflect upon. I went through many different titles, such as 'I Did Cancer ~~Wrong~~ RIGHT', 'Honouring Your Healing Path', among others, to try and capture what someone would find in these pages. Mostly, what I wanted people to get from this book is a feeling of confidence knowing that in whatever manner they go through their illness that they are honouring their personal path and to feel hopeful along the way.

As I wrote, the book evolved into something much more. I began exploring the idea that ultimately, after all of the treatments and appointments, we come to a place where we understand that loving ourselves, wholly and completely, helps us to move through this journey a little easier.

After completing my treatments I began a new path in my life – becoming the person I truly am and as a result, the most authentic 'me' emerged. After leaving my corporate job I returned to school and became a Certified Integrative Nutrition Health Coach, coaching others to achieve their wellness goals. To add to my practice, I studied and became a certified practitioner in Emotional Freedom Technique (E.F.T.) as well as Reconnective Healing®. I incorporated these modalities to help people move through any emotional blocks they may have to beginning a journey of transformation in their lives.

I also completed training with Wellspring, a cancer support organization, to lead and facilitate programs for people living with cancer and their caregivers. I currently lead groups through The Healing Journey Program and other workshops that I developed, in the areas of nutrition and energy healing. It was through my private practice, as well as my involvement at Wellspring, where I discovered that many cancer patients and caregivers struggle with the 'right' way to have cancer.

My goal in embarking on this new path was: to help people be healthy; to help people feel good about their lives; to help people transform themselves into confident, loving individuals; and to help people with cancer move beyond the illness to embrace a lifetime of wellness.

This book is a culmination of many conversations with people, observations of others and of my own personal experience with cancer. As I continued writing, the purpose of the book became clearer to me: to share insights on how to move through cancer a little easier. It covers all areas of our existence – physical, emotional, intellectual and spiritual. It begins with clearing the mind, to moving the body, to finding a spiritual purpose in your life.

It is my hope that you find this book to be helpful, whether you engage in it by simply reading it or get involved in the suggested areas of reflection. The book is laid out in a way to be able to go to any section and read on its own or start at the beginning and continue through until the end. There are stories to read along the way, things to write about, things to think about and actions to take.

Throughout these pages you will find insights, stories and ideas to reflect upon that will help you uncover your authentic self. It will lead you in the direction of finding that connection to your true self and discovering that a beautiful transformation has begun. Whether you currently have cancer, are in remission or are a caregiver for someone, this book will be helpful. Our path to healing is one in which we will always travel. My sincerest wish is that this book will help someone find an easy road.


Enjoy.

# My Story

*"Did I do cancer wrong?"*

This was a question I asked often during my treatment for non-Hodgkin's lymphoma. From those first moments I spent in a hospital bed speaking with doctors, to how I spent my days during my treatment to my post-treatment follow-up appointments. I never felt that I fit the mould of 'how to have cancer'.

*"Did I do cancer wrong?"*

What I noticed is that I didn't have the same reaction as most people. It didn't feel like a crisis to me. It didn't feel like a sentence. No tears. No anger. No 'Why me?" In a sense I knew, deep inside, that my response to having this disease was right. Not right in the sense of 'right or wrong', but rather, in being true. True for me. True for my growth. True for my healing. I understood that cancer was a catalyst for change, growth and healing. I also knew that in whatever manner I went through it, I was honouring myself.

Looking back, pre-cancer, I was intrigued by stories of how other people I knew or knew of handled this illness. Of course, I always asked the question, "If it were me, how would I handle it?" I asked the question, never expecting that I would need to find an answer. I guess it's like how I always wondered what my reaction would be if I came upon a traumatic situation, such as witnessing a car accident. Would I fall to the ground and cry or would I call 911 and then run over and help, fully composed?

What I have learned is that until you are in it, you don't know. You cannot really imagine it. I suppose if it were a play and I had the role of a person who was diagnosed, I would likely research, imagine, rehearse and then act it out. But this was not pretend. It was real. And I somehow had to figure it out.

But a funny thing happened in the beginning. An instinct took over and I knew.

Knew how to act.

Knew what to say.

Knew who to speak with.

Knew what to believe.

It was subtle, but I listened to that instinct and knew that I would do it right. And this isn't something I could have researched as a role and then rehearsed. Even if someone had shared with me the most intimate details of their own story, I could not have played that part, because as human beings we are organic and different and I could not possibly imagine how that would feel. Each of us brings to every situation our own ideas, history and experiences. I could only have cancer in my own way, in the moment.

*"Did I do cancer wrong?"*

The precise moment I knew that I wasn't doing cancer wrong came early on in the process. Due to a series of events I had to spend a couple of weeks in hospital to reduce a blood clot, resulting from a 'suspicious mass' in my upper left chest area. Within a day of being admitted, a doctor whom I knew quite well came in to see me—prior to any biopsy or diagnosis. He began apologizing for my condition. "I'm so sorry this happened to you", he cried. "Oh Linda, cancer is terrible." he went on. Maybe this was a play, after all. What dramatic role was he playing?

My response was calm and straight. I stared, eyebrows raised. "What cancer? I have not had a biopsy and there are no test results." In other words, please don't impose upon me a belief about my body, mind and spirit. The sky is not falling, Chicken Little. The definitive diagnosis had not yet been determined. I am not playing a part in your story.

In that moment, I truly believed that I was well; that I was not a victim of whatever I had going on in my body. I wasn't going to let anyone define how I should feel or what I should believe. There was no need for me to be influenced by the looks on the faces of the people around me.

In that moment, I was healthy. My life was perfect.

In that moment, I didn't have an illness. I had a wellness.

In meditation, the pause between the breaths is sometimes referred to as 'The Sacred Space'. That place where there is no thing. No reaction. No pain. No worry. No concerns. No future. No past.

During those moments, when I watched others react with drama, without knowing exactly what was happening in my body, it felt like that sacred space to me—no worries, no pain, no concerns.

*"Did I do cancer wrong?"*

Maybe I should have responded differently. Should I have bought into the idea that I had some sort of serious illness? Had I cried and panicked, looking distraught, would that have been the right thing to do? Perhaps for some, but it wasn't for me.

There is something beautiful about old movies that I just love. When I say old movies, I mean from the '40s or

'50s. I love those dramatic pauses, the hand delicately placed on the brow when someone is in distress and how simple life seemed back then. I think one of the reasons why I enjoy watching them is because, from watching them, I learn so much about my own personality. Is it my defiance that rejects the notion that I should insert those dramatic pauses in my own life? I don't know what to call it. Perhaps it's just the pragmatic part of me that rejects the drama and keeps me moving forward.

So after spending two weeks in the hospital on blood thinners to shrink the blood clot that had developed in my jugular vein from the tumor, I finally went home. A week later my family doctor called me on a Tuesday evening, around 7pm. "Linda, it's Dr. Stevens. I have news and it isn't good. The test result came back and you have cancer. It's non-Hodgkin's lymphoma." He went on to tell me about the type of lymphoma and that he was going to send a 'rush' referral to an oncologist. I stood in my kitchen, leaning over the counter, writing down whatever he told me. I hung up, looked at my husband and relayed the details.

As it turns out, they were correct. I was diagnosed with cancer at the age of 41. They were correct, but not right. They told me the results but I knew that I was the one with the result that mattered. I already knew my outcome. I listened to the voice telling me what would happen. They didn't know. I did. In an instant, I decided that I would be the director of my healing path, and everyone else? They would be my characters.

*"Did I do cancer wrong?"*

In that moment, I didn't have an illness. I had a wellness.

Not long after that call, I began what was close to a full year of appointments, tests and treatments. It was during this time I feel that my true healing occurred. Before having cancer I enjoyed a busy career, and like many people, my work life was busy and stressful. I liked the company I worked for and the people I worked with, but I knew there was something lacking for me and I was too distracted to find the time to 'figure it out'. Ironically, it wasn't until I was on medical leave for having cancer that I began reflecting on my life and listening to that inner voice telling me what to do.

This process took months and it wasn't until my last chemo treatment that I realized the answer. A friend and I were having tea and he asked me what I wanted to do with my life now. I shrugged my shoulders, the answer inside of me but still being a little lost in the question. Then he asked me this, "If you had 5 million dollars in the bank, what would you do?" Without hesitation I said, 'Help other people be healthy.'

Just like that. I knew what I wanted to do.

There were areas of my life where I was already a healer, both in my professional life and with friends and family. I was the go-to person to other people who had questions and were seeking advice. In a way that was somewhat satisfying to me, but not completely because something was still missing.

This is when my 'epiphany' happened. The moment I knew why I did cancer right. I didn't know how 'helping people be healthy' was going to look, but I had a sense of direction. Ironically, having cancer was the road there. This major shift in consciousness gave me the strength to make a major life change. So, on a micro level, I changed my life, my career, my routine—everything. On the macro level—I changed life.

Knowing that change was imminent and in a way already in progress, I went back to school. I became a certified Integrative Nutrition Health Coach at the Institute for Integrative Nutrition and continued my education beyond the school with additional courses, training, seminars and workshops. Since energy work had been helpful for me, I also took extensive training and incorporated various modes of energy healing in my practice. Merging my training with my own experience, I began facilitating programs at Wellspring Niagara, a non-profit cancer support centre. In my private practice I work with cancer patients as well as other clients who want to make changes in their lives. I have watched how illness (and/or crisis) affects people in different ways and on every level of their experience—physically, emotionally, intellectually and spiritually. I have seen what seems like a 'simple' diagnosis turn into something quite serious, and conversely, I've seen how a more advanced diagnosis can become something manageable.

*"Did I do cancer wrong?"*

Is there a right way to have cancer? What is true for you? In this book, we look at every level of our experience; our body, emotions, thoughts and spirit. What happens to our thoughts when our physical body is compromised? What are our friends and family thinking and why do they treat us differently? What's it all about? What is my purpose now? Most importantly, what can I do to help myself?

The most important lesson I learned through this journey is this: love yourself, fully and completely, so that love will be emitted toward others. It is simply that. Once we are filled with love, confidence follows. I faced a 'crisis' and learned out how to change my body, thought process, social circle and spiritual connection so that I could move forward with my healing. Much of it came during cancer; however it is an ongoing process, and one that I will continue to work on. Doing cancer 'right' has enabled me to begin a beautiful personal transformation.

> *"There is no end to education. It is not that you read a book, pass an examination, and finish with the education. The whole of life, from the moment you are born to the moment you die, is a process of learning."—Jiddu Krishnamurti*

In continuing that process of learning, my goal is to help others understand how they can help themselves, and that is because of the other important lesson I learned. It is that however I had cancer, it was the right way because it was true for me. True for how I lived my life. True because I followed the course that felt right for me. Looking back at that time, there were moments that I wondered if what I was doing or thinking or feeling or saying was right. That was all part of how to have cancer the right way. I also understood that each of those moments were gifts of growth and healing.

As I moved along through my treatments, I thought that I had missed the magical bolt of lightening which would tell me what to do. That I was comparing myself with the idea of how a person should go through cancer, rather than just being who I was in every moment. I got caught up in the role I was supposed to play—cancer patient, rather than playing the role of "me". I realize now that the bolt of lightening was happening all along. I simply needed to look up to see it.

When people ask me about my experience, I share it honestly and from my heart. I am often asked about having cancer and the 'attitude' I illustrated. People want to know how they can achieve a similar attitude to be able to move through cancer in the same way, the 'right' way.

This is why I was inspired to write this book; to share what I learned through this experience and what I gained beyond it. That by incorporating some of these insights can help people face this illness in a hopeful and inspiring way. This is an approach that shows people that they are doing cancer the right way when they are being true to themselves.

With Love,

Linda

# TRY AS YOU MIGHT, YOU CAN'T TURN OFF YOUR MIND

# Tuning In To Thoughts

*"Healing requires taking action—it is not a passive event."—Carolyn Myss*

How can understanding where your mind takes you be helpful in the healing process? It does and it really starts here. We have thoughts that are constantly cycling and swirling through our mind. We perceive things, we have ideas, we replay events; we recycle thoughts to try and make sense of them. While we are actively thinking about things, our subconscious mind is also hard at work.

Consider that your mind is like a river. Is it one that someone would go white water rafting on or is it calm and peaceful and barely moving, like a tranquil stream? Of the two, which do you think is more beneficial in healing your body?

Maybe you notice that you have been mindlessly thinking of the same thing for the past few minutes, that as you move along in your day the same annoying thought has been prominent in your mind. And perhaps it was about someone you know that said something you did not like. And because that thought about that person who said something you did not like is there, just under the surface, you notice that your irritation level has increased. That thought is guiding you. Not because it's true, but because you haven't released it. So it will stay with you, until you are aware of it, agitating you. That nasty thought will guide your actions and reactions.

When I speak with cancer patients, the idea of being aware of their thoughts has made the biggest impact for people in terms of their healing. What thoughts are stirring in their mind? When do these thoughts appear?

When we become self- aware it helps us to not only get to know ourselves better, but to identify who we are. Once we know ourselves, it is easier for us to understand what we want, how we think, how we want to be in the world and whom we want with us.

When we are first presented with a cancer diagnosis, we may begin to realize just how much we don't know ourselves. It can feel overwhelming, especially when we are faced with questions from the medical profession, friends and family.

Where does your mind take you? Are you able to pause, identify a thought that has taken over your mind and then caused a negative reaction in your body?

## SOMETHING TO TRY...

For an hour, set an alarm to go off every 20 minutes. Each time you hear the alarm, pay attention to what you are thinking about. No judgment, just notice. Do this a few times every day. Eventually, this will become automatic and you will begin noticing your thoughts while you are having them, not afterward. Awareness is key to begin the healing process.

*"Awareness is an inner quality of consciousness; it has nothing to do with closed or open eyes."—Osho*

# WRITE IT DOWN!

*"Start writing, no matter what. The water does not flow until the faucet is turned on."—Louis L'Amour*

I recall years ago coming across Julia Cameron's book called The Artist's Way. I don't know why I bought it. I may have had a longing at that time to become an artist—painter, sculptor or writer. In one of the exercises, she introduced the idea of writing morning pages as a way of accessing thoughts, owning them, moving on and creating art, characters, etc. This process of journaling has been studied and identified as a useful process on many levels. On a physical level, it can help to reduce blood pressure and increase your immune system.

In addition to physical benefits, writing and journaling offers an opportunity to get out of your mind any worrying or negative thoughts that you may be storing. When we clear our mind, removing anything that we do not need, we make room for new thoughts, ideas, and epiphanies and bring in new energy. This is important when you have cancer because it can feel isolating. While there are friends and family that try to understand what you may be going through, they may not be able to truly comprehend your thoughts and feelings.

In order for this to be successful, I learned early on that you need to take the 'perfectionism' out of the process. Grammar and punctuation are not the focus. A scribble here and a scribble there are just part of the flow. You can write in complete sentences, point-form or jot down a list of words. You can doodle, draw an image or sketch something meaningful to you. Any way that you journal is the right way if you are managing to express your emotions and experience peace.

Here is an example of what journaling may look like early on:

*"Oh my god, it's so early. I can't believe I am up this early. I have nothing to say. I just want to go back to sleep. Now I have to pee. Gotta find my slippers. Why am I doing this anyway? Supposedly I am going to find some sort of enlightenment. Maybe I'll make soup today since Janice had to cancel our coffee date. That's the second time. Hmm, wonder what's up. Maybe it's because I'm too negative about my hair. Too bad. I have cancer. I can complain as much as I want. I have to pee. Am I done yet? How long is this exercise supposed to take? What else. What else. What else can I write? I need carrots for my soup. I don't want to go out. People stare at my hair. Or lack of it. My wig itches. This sucks. I'm tired. Maybe I should try to sleep more. Ok, just a few more paragraphs. I'm supposed to commit to writing.*

*"I could draw. The book says drawing can be part of journaling. I suck at drawing. I can only manage stick people. Ok here goes. Ok, this is kind of funny. What are these stick people doing? I feel crappy. My tummy hurts. Maybe I should make tea. Ginger is probably best. These drugs are wrecking my digestion. I hate them. Only 6 rounds of chemo left. Woohoo for me!! Sarcasm isn't working. Right, gotta change my thoughts. After six more rounds of chemo, I'll be done and ready to move ahead. Better."*

After time it becomes, your writing becomes focused and clear. The emotions that you express help you bring in peace and healing.

An example may look like this:

"Had a great sleep and feel rested. Good thing since I am off to another chemo treatment today. Well, hopefully today if my blood numbers are good. I feel strong so I think I'm good to go. I wonder if I'll have Alice as my nurse today. Love her. I wonder if she started yoga like I suggested. She likely needs the stretch but more importantly, I think she needs the meditation that goes with it. She has a million things going on in her life. No wonder I find her to be distracted at times.

"My mind is relaxed and calm today. This feels good. I'm happy that I'm able to have some peace. Finally. I finally feel that I'm learning the lessons I need to move forward for myself. This process is all about me. The appointments and the self-care that I'm doing are helping me to survive. I knew I needed to change my life, but I didn't have the courage. I should write about that today during chemo. Having the courage to change. Having the strength to move forward with my life. This illness has become my full-time job. How did I fit it all in before?

"Had a wonderful dream last night. I was flying over an ocean. The colour of the water is what I remember most. I don't know if I could find that hue of blue. There were moments that I barely skimmed the water. It was warm and I expected it to be cool. Weird. I wonder what dreaming about water means. I'll have to research that.

"I'm going to make some gluten free energy bars before I go. Mmmm, the pumpkin ones that I love."

Studies that have been conducted on various groups who journal, note that stress levels decrease and immune function increases when they are journaling about their thoughts and emotions. When you have an accelerated amount of stress and keep it in, your body reacts by increasing the stress hormones, which, among other things, affects your immune function. When you are given an avenue to release that stress, you feel happier, calmer and in control.

There is a quote by Marlene Schiwy that partly states "Keeping a journal does not simply mean recording external facts of your life from one day to the next... Journal writing is a process of vital reflection that plunges you below the surface of your life to its psychic roots. When you are writing at that deeper level, your life itself changes."

A common response to the idea of journaling is the feeling that you need to be an author to gain the benefits from journaling. Remember that you aren't writing a best seller. You simply want to rid your mind of the busy thoughts, the worrying thoughts and the thoughts that keep cycling around. You can write in full sentences, point form or doodle. It all works. It is all the 'right' way.

The writing exercise will help you to begin writing, without having to try and think about what you want to write about. Give it a try!

## TIME FOR REFLECTION

If you like, you can reflect upon the following statements and questions and either meditate on or write about them in a journal.

1. I am not what I have done. I am what I have overcome.

2. If I had absolutely no restrictions, how would I spend my time each day?

3. "Reflect upon your present blessings of which every man has many- not on your past misfortunes, of which all men have some." (Charles Dickens)

4. "Health is the greatest gift, contentment the greatest wealth, faithfulness the best relationship." (Buddha)

5. The top 3 things I need to change right now for my healing are...

6. Select a poem, read it and write about how it makes you feel.

7. Recall a favourite vacation and write about all of the details of the trip; where you went, who was with you, describe what you saw and how you felt.

8. If I could have a 'do-over' for a situation that happened in my life, which would it be and what would I do differently?

9. Write a letter to your future self.

# MEDITATION

When I mention the idea of beginning a meditation practice to people, the most common response I hear is either "I can't do it" or "I've tried it. It doesn't work for me." If I could take just a moment here, I want to share with you how well it does work. And it can work for everyone—including you.

When you think of meditation, you may conjure up a vision of a Buddhist monk, sitting cross-legged with his hands resting in his lap, eyes closed. There is a feeling of serenity in that image, and then comes the feeling that it looks too difficult.

The way I describe meditation to the groups I lead is that meditation is not about getting to a destination or being someplace at the end; it's about the unfolding that happens along the way. There is no need to worry about where you should be going and what is supposed to happen when you get there. It's about observing. Being in the moment. Noticing. First meditate and then see where you end up.

The Buddhist Center website describes meditation like this. " Meditation is a means of transforming the mind. Meditation practices are techniques that encourage and develop concentration, clarity, emotional positivity, and a calm seeing of the true nature of things. By engaging with a particular meditation practice you learn the patterns and habits of your mind, and the practice offers a means to cultivate new, more positive ways of being. With regular work and patience these nourishing, focused states of mind can deepen into profoundly peaceful and energized states of mind. Such experiences can have a transformative effect and can lead to a new understanding of life."

There is much research on the benefits of meditation. Studies have been conducted which show improvement in blood pressure, immune system and sleep patterns, among other things. It can actually help your body's stress level by helping to reduce cortisol levels.

## SOMETHING TO TRY... GUIDED IMAGERY

To begin, sit comfortably in a quiet area. Close your eyes.

Scan your body and notice if there is tension in any area. We commonly hold tension in the jaw, shoulders and neck. By using your breath, with each exhalation release any tension in those areas. This is not something that is forced. Simply relax, breath and release.

Imagine that you are in a natural, relaxing setting, like a forest or a beach. When you are doing this, really imagine each detail—colour, sounds, smells and temperature. Take your time with this step because this will help you to feel more relaxed. Since it is your image, use whatever details you like, even if it seems fantastical. Go ahead. There is no judgment here in your guided meditation.

You can imagine anything at all. What is most important is that it is a relaxing setting where you can maintain a feeling of stillness in your mind.

Once there, begin to empty your mind of any thoughts of past or future, events that took place or what is to come, conversations that happened or ones that will. If you notice your mind wandering, simply refocus on the details of the setting—colours, sounds, etc. Having a detailed image to begin with will help you get there more easily.

Empty your mind of thoughts. One way to achieve this is to imagine a grey cloud in your mind, where nothing resides. If you notice your mind wandering, gently come back to your imagery of a grey cloud. You may want to focus on a sound in that is in your setting; perhaps if there is a bird there, to help ground you in that setting.

Stay in this place for as long as you like. When you are ready to complete the meditation, begin to make small movements with your hands and feet, while bringing your awareness to the sounds around you. Open your eyes.

This process allows you to focus on images and sounds, without your mind being filled with thoughts. You are simply seeing the surroundings, feeling the area, and hearing sounds—a bird or a wave from the ocean.

## SOMETHING TO TRY... LOVING KINDNESS MEDITATION

This is a beautiful meditation with the focus on feeling feeling pure love. In it you are feeling love, directing love and experiencing love. This meditation has many variations, but mainly it is to direct loving kindness to yourself, then to others you know and finally to the rest of the planet. The script below is one that you can use. Don't worry about doing it wrong. It isn't necessary to memorize it in order to do the meditation 'right'. As long as you have the main phrases and your intention is clear, you are doing it right.

This particular version is from Jack Kornfield and can be found on his website: jackkornfield.com.

## LOVING KINDNESS MEDITATION

This meditation uses words, images, and feelings to evoke a loving kindness and friendliness toward oneself and others. With each recitation of the phrases, we are expressing an intention, planting the seeds of loving wishes over and over in our heart.

*With a loving heart as the background, all that we attempt, all that we encounter will open and flow more easily. You can begin the practice of loving kindness by meditating for fifteen or twenty minutes in a quiet place. Let yourself sit in a comfortable fashion. Let your body rest and be relaxed. Let your heart be soft. Let go of any plans or preoccupations.*

*Begin with yourself. Breathe gently, and recite inwardly the following traditional phrases directed toward our own well-being. You begin with yourself because without loving yourself it is almost impossible to love others.*

*May I be filled with loving kindness.*

*May I be safe from inner and outer dangers.*

*May I be well in body and mind.*

*May I be at ease and happy.*

*As you repeat these phrases, picture yourself as you are now, and hold that image in a heart of loving kindness. Or perhaps you will find it easier to picture yourself as a young and beloved child. Adjust the words and images in any way you wish. Create the exact phrases that best open your heart of kindness.*

*Repeat these phrases over and over again, letting the feelings permeate your body and mind. Practice this meditation for a number of weeks, until the sense of* loving kindness for yourself grows.

Be aware that this meditation may at times feel mechanical or awkward. It can also bring up feelings contrary to loving kindness, feelings of irritation and anger. If this happens, it is especially important to be patient and kind toward yourself, allowing whatever arises to be received in a spirit of friendliness and kind affection. When you feel you have established some stronger sense of loving kindness for yourself, you can then expand your meditation to include others. After focusing on yourself for five or ten minutes, choose a benefactor, someone in your life who has loved and truly cared for you. Picture this person and carefully recite the same phrases:

May you be filled with loving kindness.

May you be safe from inner and outer dangers.

May you be well in body and mind.

May you be at ease and happy.

Let the image and feelings you have for your benefactor support the meditation. Whether the image or feelings are clear or not does not matter. In meditation they will be subject to change. Simply continue to plant the seeds of loving wishes, repeating the phrases gently no matter what arises.

Expressing gratitude to our benefactors is a natural form of love. In fact, some people find loving kindness for themselves so hard, they begin their practice with a benefactor. This too is fine. The rule in loving kindness practice is to follow the way that most easily opens your heart.

When loving kindness for your benefactor has

*developed, you can gradually begin to include other people in your meditation. Picturing each beloved person, recite inwardly the same phrases, evoking a sense of loving kindness for each person in turn.*

*After this you can include others: Spend some time wishing well to a wider circle of friends. Then gradually extend your meditation to picture and include community members, neighbors, people everywhere, animals, all beings, the whole earth.*

*Finally, include the difficult people in your life, even your enemies, wishing that they too may be filled with loving kindness and peace. This will take practice. But as your heart opens, first to loved ones and friends, you will find that in the end you won't want to close it anymore.*

Loving kindness can be practiced anywhere. You can use this meditation in traffic jams, in buses, and on airplanes. As you silently practice this meditation among people, you will come to feel a wonderful connection with them – the power of loving kindness. It will calm your mind and keep you connected to your heart.

I began meditating shortly after I was diagnosed with cancer. It was difficult for me, however I knew that the benefit far outweighed the discomfort. In the beginning my mind raced, I was frustrated and I couldn't sit still for very long. However, the more I meditated, the easier it became. Today, I use guided meditation when I am facilitating groups as a way to model how peaceful one can feel from the practice of meditation. Participants note that they feel more relaxed, are open to thoughts and because of this are willing to try it at home.

I hope you will too.

*"Your vision will become clear only when you look into your heart. Who looks inside awakens." - Carl Yung*

# EMOTION IS MOTION

# Make Wellness Your Full Time Job

Your life is different now. You have cancer. To think that you will go about your routine the same way as before is no longer realistic. Accepting is a good place to begin. It's all about you. Your body needs your full attention.

When you are first diagnosed, after the initial shock dissipates, a lot of thoughts go through your mind. You begin to realize the time commitment that is ahead of you and you consider how you will fit your medical appointments and treatments into your existing life. This does not even include any other appointments and coping skills you want to incorporate—massage, meditation, exercise, and so on. Your pre–cancer life is the only schedule you know and understand, but you want to get this right and fit everything in that you need. Eventually you come to understand that your way of life, as you know it, is going to be different. It needs to be different. When you engage in the belief that you are a priority, it makes the healing process that much easier.

Are you doing cancer wrong if you don't make your healing a priority? No, not at all. Having cancer is a lot of work and sometimes people just don't feel like doing a lot of the extras. You may find it easier to incorporate a couple of self–care techniques while you are in treatment and do only those things. After your treatments have ended you can add to the existing complement of self–care tools. This is a perfectly acceptable way to do it.

Part of the struggle I notice with many patients, is their desire to control how their illness fits into their lives. It would be much easier if they could have cancer on their own terms and in their own way. They often feel the need to keep up appearances, maintaining the life they had while trying to fit in doing what they need to do to get better.

To prioritize your healing work, it needs to be considered first, before any other invitations or events. Early on in your diagnosis, you will likely be overwhelmed with calls and emails because everyone will want to help and be there for you. People will want to take you places, come for a visit and drop off food. Since you are likely still in a state of shock, you welcome the attention. You also want to continue doing all of the things you did before—go to your book club meeting, take your son to baseball practice, make cookies for the church bake sale.

It may be a good practice after each invitation to stop and ask yourself, "Am I making my healing a priority in any of these scenarios?" Taking care of some of our regular tasks can help in our healing. It can feel empowering when you can continue doing things that you typically do. It feels good to keep up with your routine. You might question whether you are allowing them to get in the way, perhaps distracting you. When are you adding in rest, meditation, journaling or gentle yoga?

Having cancer can be an opportunity to develop a new way of life, one that is aligned with your healing path. Beginning this journey will help you to develop a new you. Inevitably you are a changed person. Who you are, what you think, how you live, relationships you have – all of that is changing. And will change for the better.

Give some thought as to how you will prioritize what is important in your new life. Many people I speak with use a calendar of some sort—paper or electronic. They schedule everything they need to do for themselves first and all of the other events around that schedule, and once it's in the calendar they commit to it. I recall a member of one of my groups mentioning that she used a day timer. She scheduled time for yoga, meditation and journaling through the week. When she would receive an invitation that could possibly conflict with her self-care time, rather than canceling it, she would move it to another time in the day. If it didn't fit anywhere else, she would decline the invitation.

## TIME FOR REFLECTION

If you like, you can reflect upon the following statements or questions and either meditate on or write about them in a journal.

1. Make a list of your current activities and note how much time in a day you spend doing each one.

2. Looking at the list, are there activities that you would like to do that are missing?

3. How can you implement these missing activities from into your life?

4. What obstacles do you feel could get in the way?

# You're Going to Be Tired! Honour It!

Ah sleep! The joy of laying your head down on a pillow, closing your eyes and allowing your mind to drift off to dreamland. If only you did not feel like you needed to sleep all day long. One of the more common side effects of cancer treatments is fatigue. The Mayo Clinic states that some of the causes of fatigue are the cancer itself (taxing your biological system), the treatment (chemo or radiation), pain, emotions, lack of sleep and poor nutrition. Lacking energy and feeling sleepy adds to the frustration of having cancer.

When you are relaxing your body is restoring, but how do you get rest that helps you feel as though you have rested? You may feel that sleep isn't what you need, but simply a physical rest. Take time to sit and relax as often as needed. You may also notice that you feel tired when you are around people, using your energy to take part in conversations, (both in speaking and to focus on what is being said). It is also acceptable to take a break from seeing people.

If you are looking to increase your energy level, here are some suggestions:

1. Try a few gentle yoga poses. There are a couple of things helping - movement and breathing. Moderate exercise can improve your mobility and energy levels. You can join a class or buy a DVD to use at home.

2. Hydrate, hydrate, hydrate. Increasing your hydration helps increase your level of energy and also helps to remove energy-zapping toxins from your system.

3. Take a nap. Make it a habit to sleep, even if you aren't sleepy. If you begin the habit of resting throughout the day, your body will become accustomed to it and you will feel more energized from the small breaks.

4. Eat fresh foods and avoid the processed ones. Fresh fruits and vegetables contain enzymes that help you to digest foods easily. When your digestive system is working properly your system is not taxed and you will have more energy.

5. Maintain a cooler temperature in your bedroom. When the temperature is above 20 degrees Celsius or 68 degrees Fahrenheit, our bodies become warm and we have a tendency to wake up or have an uncomfortable sleep.

# LET THOSE TEARS FLOW!

Allowing yourself to feel and express emotions is essential to your healing. This place that you are in now is unlike any place you have been before. It is important not to tuck away emotions deep inside your body. This can result in creating unhealthy stress that your body does not need.

Sara relayed her experience with me and it resonated on so many levels. With her permission, I am honoured to share it here.

## SARA'S STORY

*"From the moment I heard the words, 'You have cancer', my eyes welled up with tears and they began to flow down my cheeks. Every memory from my life and moment that I lived flashed across my mind. I was aware of all of it. Something took over and the floodgates opened. I understood on some level that a transformation was beginning, but it felt so big and I was so overwhelmed that I released it all in that instant.*

*I came here from another country and was a young woman during a time when women were considered mostly to bear of children and keep a good home. My mother was one, my grandmother as well, and all the other women in my life maintained a similar existence. Everyone went about their day, kept to themselves and when emotions arose, we rarely let them be seen by others.*

*When I met and married Frederick, I knew that my life would be different. He was kind, quiet and genuinely interested in me, not only as a possible wife and mother of our children, but in me as a woman. We had a good life together. It was modest, but we managed to raise our children, gave them an education and all of the things they needed. Well, they may not agree because I'm certain, as children, they would have wanted more toys and maybe a fancy vacation.*

*Frederick and I spent our years together as most couples do; we became part of our community, socialized with our family and friends, celebrated birthdays, anniversaries and holidays. We were also there for each other during difficult times, the loss of a job, a car accident, the death of someone close.*

*At that moment of diagnosis sitting in the doctor's office, in a flash, each of those memories appeared in my mind. It was like I could recall each one and I relived them in an instant. I felt every feeling I had during those moments– joy, love, laughter, sadness, pain and loss. I wondered what it all meant now. How would this diagnosis fit into the lives of people around me? Would it change the memories?*

*After hearing the diagnosis from my doctor, he excused himself and Frederick and I sat still for a moment. When my tears kept flowing, Frederick was at a loss. He didn't know what to say and I think said what most people would, 'It'll be ok. Don't cry. Don't worry.'*

*But I needed those tears. Crying helped me to feel real. The tears were also for so many times in my life where I wanted to cry, but didn't. I realize that I needed to let them out in order for the healing to begin. I didn't want to stop the tears from flowing. Healing for me wasn't just about surgery. It was a process of allowing, of honouring myself.*

Later, when Frederick asked me if I felt sad about my situation, I told him that I didn't. The tears weren't about regret or fear, but rather I felt that there was a cleansing taking place. After reassuring him that I was okay, we gathered my protocol and information from the doctor and left the appointment with a plan in hand.

All through having cancer, I continued to allow the tears to flow whenever I needed them. For fear of alarming Frederick, I didn't let him see me, or anyone else for that matter, but I cried. And afterward, I always felt better. Empty. Empty in a good way. And somehow that allowed me to feel happier because I made room inside for happiness."

"What soap is for the body, tears are for the soul."
—Jewish Proverb

# ACCEPT HELP!

For some, it is important to maintain a certain persona when they have cancer. A way of presenting themselves to others that says they are not weak and a victim of their circumstance. Rather than embracing their friends and family's support, they refuse any offers of help, not taking heed of people who just love them and want to be there in any way they can. Am I doing cancer wrong by not accepting help from others? No, it is not wrong, but a good question to ask might be, "Why aren't you?"

## ED'S STORY

*I met Ed when he was in remission. I can only describe him as being 'stubborn'. I say that lovingly because Ed, at 58 years old, having had Stage 2 prostrate cancer, will shake his head and laugh at himself about his stubbornness. At the time of his diagnosis, he owned his own landscaping business and had one full-time and one seasonal employee. Having the business for almost 20 years, he had gained a loyal client base. Many of his customers felt like old friends to Ed. He knew them well, along with their families and he would hear of their lives and events like graduations and weddings.*

*After meeting with his medical team, Ed opted to treat the cancer with whatever was medically required. He also decided that he was going to continue working through his treatments. He was told that he was being stubborn and that he should be taking care of himself, but at the time Ed did not feel that way at all. He just wanted to carry on as a 'regular' guy.*

His wife, Becky, felt differently; she was fearful. The word 'cancer' is a negative word to her. There was too much that was unknown and she was afraid of the unknown. She and a few close friends of Ed's tried every which way to convince him to stop working, focus on his health and rely on his staff. However Ed couldn't do it. He felt that if he were to slow down, even the slightest bit, that it would be a sign of weakness. Also, Ed didn't want to 'look' sick. He felt that if he continued with his usual routine, people wouldn't treat him differently.

Shortly after beginning his treatments Ed started feeling tired and was struggling to keep up, but he kept working a very physical job. Digging, cutting, pruning, not to mention booking appointments, working on quotes and coordinating supplies: he did it all.

After a couple of weeks of having treatments, Ed suffered a physical breakdown. He became dizzy and weak almost daily. On one particular day, Ed fell over and nearly fainted when he was at home. Becky was scared and stayed with him constantly, tending to his needs. She made soup, tea and filled hot water bottles, but more importantly, she became Ed's guard dog. She shielded him from phone calls and anything related to business. She spoke with his employees and together, they figured it out and ran the business for Ed.

The day Ed nearly fell over changed him. He realized just how fragile his health was and even worse, that he was disregarding it. He also realized that if he continued on this path, his healing would take much, much longer. Ed eased away from work, but stayed involved by directing his staff and answering calls. Becky stepped in and took over the coordination of jobs. Ed handed over control of some of the business *and as a result, he gained control of his life back.*

*What also changed for him was that he began to take charge of his healing. He researched healthy recipes. He joined a support group. He started going to a gentle yoga class. By embracing the fact that he had cancer, allowed him to let go and accept help. Ed realized that he was not a weak man for accepting help, but rather a strong man for knowing how to take care of himself. This is what allowed him to begin to own his healing path.*

Part of that healing was about knowing when to accept help. As much as Ed tried to turn people away, he needed them in the end. This is true for everyone. What is it that you need in order to move through your treatments more easily? Are you willing to live differently? How can you surrender to the help of others without surrendering yourself?

Once you know what areas you need help with, ask! Simply ask for help. In my work with cancer patients, I have met many people who have groups of friends, family or coworkers offering to help with anything. When they offer, they mean it. They want to help because they feel helpless and this is the one thing that they feel will help you get better. They will do whatever they can to be there for you. To have help preparing meals, being driven places, having someone to chat with, all go a long way in your healing.

How is this doing cancer right? You are being true to your needs. It is okay to do things on your own, but when you have help life is a little easier. It builds a feeling of community. It allows other people to feel as though they are helping. Ed's story could be anyone's story. We have strength in knowing when to ask for help and accepting it.

## TIME FOR REFLECTION

If you like, you can reflect upon the following statements and questions and either meditate on or write about them in a journal.

1. Where in my life am I most helpful to others?

2. What needs to change in my mind and spirit in order for me to accept help from others?

3. If I could imagine a perfect day, just for me, doing whatever I like, describe the day.

4. If someone I loved was in need, how would I want to help him or her? What can I ask for from others?

*"Generosity is giving more than you can...pride is taking less than you need. "—Anonymous*

# TALK IT OUT. IT HELPS TO SHARE

Having the love and support of your friends and family is invaluable when you have cancer. However, their understanding of how you feel is influenced by the fact that they aren't going through what you are going through. They are likely feeling the stress of doing or saying the 'wrong' thing, because they can't identify with what you are experiencing and are fearful of upsetting you. When you are sharing your feelings, you may get a response like, 'Keep you chin up', when what you really need is someone who understands what you are going through and who will listen when you are sharing your stories and expressing your needs.

Finding a support group is essential in the healing process. It's helpful to know that you are not alone and that other people experience similar feelings. It can help you to feel like you are not crazy to think the things you are thinking. A support group has a leader with experience leading the dialogue. The conversations are structured, safe and honest. There is a theme at each session to begin the dialogue. Another helpful aspect of a group is that other members who have gone through a similar situation, may have a suggestion that can help you in your healing. At the very least, they can listen, nod and offer an understanding ear.

Another benefit is the sharing of information, community resources, books to read and treatment information. A support group doesn't replace formal counseling and usually the expert facilitating the group will be able to identify someone who needs further support and will make a recommendation, if necessary.

A study conducted with women who had metastatic breast cancer (1989, The Lancet October) showed that women who participated in a support group lived approximately 18 months longer than those women who did not participate. The focus of the support group encompassed living life fully, improving communication with family and doctors, facing death and expressing emotion.

A support group can also be useful in offering the simplest of tips. I recall that a woman at one of the groups I attended, Nancy, shared how she could not handle the nausea after her chemo treatments. Although she took the medication recommended by the physician, it still was not helping and she was having a lot of problems. Another woman from the group shared that she makes her own ginger tea (hot water, a chunk of ginger and a touch of honey) and that it worked for her. When we met for the following session, Nancy told us that she had given it a try and found that it helped her.

One other benefit to finding a group is how it can alleviate stress placed on a caregiver. A gentleman I met, Rick, mentioned that he knew he was causing his wife stress. He noticed that she was more irritable and tired since his diagnosis. He told me that he shared his thoughts and feelings with her all the time and she didn't always know what to say or do. Rick said that once he found a group, he began speaking and sharing his thoughts with them. He soon observed that his wife was more relaxed.

After talking about what he discovered with his wife, he understood the pressure he was placing on her to be a caregiver and his sounding board. She told him that she was so worried about saying the wrong thing that she would bottle it up and she became more agitated. Having a group for Rick to attend has helped her immensely. An interesting thing happened; seeing the difference it made for Rick, his wife then sought a caregiver support group to help her as well.

"Stay with friends who support you in these. Talk with them about sacred texts, and how you are doing, and how they are doing, and keep your practices together."—Rumi (1207 - 1273)

# YOUR BODY IS YOUR TEMPLE

# You're Going to Eat What?!

> "The doctor of the future will give no medication, but will interest his patients in the care of the human frame, diet and in the cause and prevention of disease."—Thomas A Edison

This is a story that illustrates what I came to understand about the need people have to find comfort in their journey, even in the smallest things.

## Linda's Story

*I had quite the eye-opening experience during my chemo treatments when it came to eating and nourishment, and I got an added life lesson on judgment, too. The hospital where I was treated was a 50-minute drive from home so when I had appointments and treatments, I went prepared. And prepared I was. I brought my own bottle of alkaline water, a healthy lunch, a thermos of tea and a book of crossword puzzles. I also packed an extra sweater in case I was cold and a journal for any inspirational moments I wanted to capture. (I rarely had any).*

*The room in which I had chemo was large and accommodated many patients. Our chairs were those comfortable hospital 'lazy-boy' style chairs. They weren't spaced very far apart so this gave me an opportunity to look around and see what other patients had with them.*

*Typically, I would be there for about 6—8 hours; the day was long and many patients came and went. They also brought their own snacks and drinks. I also noticed that the snacks were on the opposite end of the spectrum. As I sat and unpacked my homemade quinoa salad with roasted organic vegetables and home made gluten-free, sugar free biscotti, I watched others as they opened bags of chips, ate doughnuts and drank some form of cola.*

*You're eating what? Was the question I asked silently in my head. Why? Why would they do that? How could they treat their bodies so poorly? Who is in charge here? Take that away!*

*Of course, I was sitting in judgment of them. I recognize that now and really, who was I to decide how people should be eating? Certainly, there is much evidence to support how a healthy diet helps our bodies in the healing process, but I need to call myself out on this one. The one thing I was not seeing at the time was that it was comfort people were seeking, and, in part, that they were getting it from their food. I understand this thinking, having battled my own emotional eating disorder.*

*Perhaps they were hurting, sad and maybe a little fearful. Maybe eating those foods and eating for comfort helped them to feel like their normal selves. Maybe, by eating foods they would have otherwise avoided when they didn't have cancer, a person could hold onto the idea that they didn't have it at all. And just maybe, in their mind, the attitude of 'screw you, cancer' was prevalent. And although they were sitting in a room full of scarf-wrapped heads and people in distress, that they could somehow feel 'normal'.*

I can't argue with that, and in fact I no longer judge it. It is the reason I do the work that I do now. It is certainly my wish that people take care of themselves in every way possible; but really, if someone wants a coffee with extra cream and two sugars because by having a cup, it will give them an emotional lift, go ahead! Without knowing them, I couldn't possibly understand the reason, but I can have foster compassion.

Know that it is okay to stray with your diet once in a while. If you are following a specific dietary regime that is working well, then stick with it, but you can feel overwhelmed by all of the information that is available. When your physical body is not well, your mind and spirit are in a weakened state, too. You can feel as though you are having cancer the wrong way if you have a cup of coffee. Perhaps you have decided that your treatment day is the day you have something on the naughty list!

It's okay to stray. You have permission to do what you need to do to feel better. When you are ready, you can get back on track. What I tell my clients who are trying to lose weight and clean up their eating is that if they deviate from their plan, rather than beating themselves up for the rest of the day and perhaps into the next one, just start right now. Make right now your new start. There is no point in discounting the great work you have completed thus far.

Let's look at the 'right now'. Right now, your body is in need of the best nutrition you can give it. By making a few changes, like reducing sugar and eating whole foods, it will help your body right now. Some of the more popular lifestyles that people adopt during cancer are: vegetarian/vegan, raw and organic. There are many more, but these are written about frequently in conjunction with any cancer dialogue.

It is important to stress that whatever manner of diet you choose, own the decision for yourself. Align your mind with your body. You will find that friends or family will read something about a life changing super-food or have spoken to someone about a particular diet and they want you to be aware of it. You know what is best for you. Trust your instinct. Honour that! Be true to what works for you.

*"The way you think, the way you behave, the way you eat, can influence your life by 30 to 50 years."*—Deepak Chopra

## Time for Reflection

If you like, you can reflect upon the following questions and either meditate on or write about them in a journal.

1. Think about your diet before being diagnosed with cancer. How did that diet fit into your life? If it didn't, what changes have you thought about making?

2. Think about how you eat now, after being diagnosed. Have you made changes? If so, what have you changed?

3. What is your ideal lifestyle when it comes to eating? What does that look like? What would a sample menu be?

4. Which eating plan feels right for you, in this moment? How can you implement it?

# Every Once in a While, You Have to Change the Music!

There is something to be said about the effect that music has on our physical body, not to mention our mind and spirit. I listened to a lot of sacred music as I was going through treatments. It was calming, beautiful, inspirational and loving.

However every so often, I felt edgy—not on edge, but fearless, strong, a 'conquer the world' attitude, especially when I would think back to that day in the hospital bed with the very apologetic doctor and my response of "What cancer?" It was during those moments that I would turn on music that helped bring me back to that attitude, back to that part of me that is fearless and strong. The music that helped was anything that brought me to a time when I was happy, giddy, in love, silly or reminded me of old friends. It was nostalgic. You know that line 'dance like nobody is watching'? Well, I did and it felt AWESOME.

Laughter has a similar effect on the body. When you laugh your body moves, which means your muscles are moving. Your breathing alters and you become breathless (moving the stale air from your lungs) and take in a deep breath, bringing in fresh, clean new air. Your pulse rate increases, bringing changes to your heart. It feels good.

## SOMETHING TO TRY...

1. Play music that makes you want to scream out loud as you sing along and then shake it up. Move your body, however much you can. Just move. Sway. Jump. Swing. Twirl. Let your body move naturally to the rhythm. Enjoy!

2. Watch movies or TV shows that make you laugh out loud. Do this daily. Laugh so much and so hard that tears pour down your face and your cheek muscles begin to hurt.

# RESEARCHING THE INTERNET

*"Getting information off the Internet is like taking a drink from a fire hydrant"—Mitchell Kapor*

We are so attached to information, aren't we? That Google search engine provides mounds of information, details and resources that help us move along our lives so much easier. However, if we aren't careful, that lovely, helpful search engine can become a flying monster that swoops in, picks us up and carries us to the land of 'I'm freaking out over here'.

## DUNCAN'S STORY

*Duncan called me one day after his sister gave him my business card. We set up an appointment and he came to see me.*

*"Yeah, I have cancer. My sister thinks that I should talk to someone. But I'm not crazy or anything."*

*"Great, that's good to know. What does she think you need to talk about?"*

*"I'm driving everyone crazy because I don't know what's going to happen, and I keep reading the Internet, and I think I have every symptom, and I don't know what to do about it. I knew it was time to do something when I was convinced that my toenails were turning a shade of green after reading something about side effects."*

*Duncan's story is typical for so many people who are anxious about what treatments will be like and, more importantly, if will they work. It is natural to feel anxious and wonder, but when it takes you to a place of anxiety and fear it's time to find help for yourself. I began working with Duncan using Emotional Freedom Technique to help reduce his anxiety. When we began, we worked on his worry that the treatments that he was going to receive would be painful, take a long time and worse, that they may not get rid of the cancer.*

*After a session of working together on his fear of pain, Duncan was prepared to address what he was truly feeling at our following session: fear of dying. Duncan admitted that it was all he could think about. He was afraid to burden anyone so he didn't talk about it. Instead he spent time researching the Internet looking for treatments, statistics and stories to try and calm himself down. For Duncan, the reverse was happening. The more he read, the worse it became and the higher his anxiety level spiked.*

*Together, we worked on two issues: his need to know and his fear of dying. After two more sessions, his anxiety level dropped. He still thought about the cancer and also about the possibility of dying, but when he did he wasn't as anxious. Duncan felt that he could talk about it and, in fact, wanted to share how he was feeling. Rather than speaking with his family, he began attending a cancer support group so that he could share with others and gain support.*

Duncan's story is similar to so many stories of people with cancer. The desire to feel reassured drives people to search for answers. Many people feel scared, alone and are worried that their thoughts will be a burden to others.

One suggestion to remember while researching information is to use discernment. Before accessing information, ask yourself what information do you require in this moment. As you search, keep these questions in mind:

*Are you reviewing a reliably sourced site?*

*Is the information evidence based?*

*How will this information serve you?*

# BELIEVE THAT YOUR TREATMENT PLAN IS RIGHT FOR YOU.

*"A good decision is based on knowledge and not numbers."—Plato*

Sometimes attitude can make all of the difference. There is a substantial amount of media coverage surrounding cancer, treatment options and therapies, however one area that does not receive a lot of coverage is how believing in what you are doing can have an impact your healing.

From a conventional treatment perspective, there is chemotherapy, radiation and surgery. Additionally, you will also consider other modalities such as diet, exercise, massage, mediation, vitamins and supplements. Making these decisions can feel overwhelming and confusing. When we are presented with too many choices, we may ask the question "What exactly is the right choice for me?" or "Am I doing it the right way?"

Let's look at an analogy of needing to purchase a new furnace for your house. How would you go about this task? Often it begins with research, such as speaking to others to get an opinion on model, style, price and installer. You may also research what type would be best for your home. You may even read a few reviews after you've narrowed down a few brands.

Once you make your final decision, you can feel confident in knowing that you made the best selection for your home, at that time, based on all of the available information you had.

It is not very different when making a decision for your treatment plan. After you are diagnosed, most often you will speak to a doctor to see what they recommend, do a little research of your own and then use your intuition to decide which route is best for you. Whichever plan you choose, it's the right plan for you.

When you doubt your decisions or feel uncertain about your treatment plan, it can be detrimental to your healing. It can create stress, which can lead to lack of sleep, agitation and irritability. How can this mindset possibly feel healing?

Attitude can make a difference. When you approach the plan with optimism and joy, it will make a difference to your outcome. Your mind is aligned with your body in welcoming the treatment plan. This positive approach will make a difference in how your body reacts, such as having fewer side effects. Think about it in terms of being required to do something that you don't enjoy. Do you walk toward it slowly, hunched over? Or do you skip there with joy and excitement?

I have one last comment concerning my own experience. On the day I went for my first chemo treatment, I sat in the waiting room listening for my name to be called. As I waited, my oncologist came to find me. She sat across from me, looked directly into my eyes and told me that one of the reasons she took my case was because of my attitude. She continued to tell me that of all of her patients, the people with a positive outlook do better than those that do not. That meant a lot to me and I have never forgotten it.

Here are a few tips to help you lessen the doubt and move forward with confidence:

First, trust that you know best. You are constantly learning your likes and dislikes. It is how you grow as an individual. While you may not have had the experience of making decisions about cancer, you have made decisions about what is best for you for most of your lifetime. Trust that. How did you make important decisions for yourself before cancer? Using that same process will be helpful.

Second, know that you can change your mind if you begin to feel that what you are doing isn't right for you. This is also part of our learning process. It is okay to make a mistake. It's going to happen in your lifetime and making them when you have cancer can happen, too.

Lastly, have no regrets. When you are making a decision, you are making it at a time when you have all of the information in front of you. You cannot possibly know that something else is going to come along in a few months that will change your mind. You can only choose based on the information you have in the moment. If you begin regretting your decision as soon as you make it, you will feel like you are constantly losing your mind.

*"Nobody can give you wiser advice than yourself"*
—*Cicero*

# MOVEMENT

There are numerous benefits to incorporating some form of exercise when you have cancer. The website cancer.org lists some of these as helping to improve balance and flexibility, lowering the risk of becoming anxious, depressed and tired, improving blood flow to reduce clots, and improving quality of life.

There are some gentle movement techniques that, along with incorporating specific breathing patterns, can feel energizing. Many of these classes can be found at local community centres in your area.

Here are three of them.

YOGA – There are many styles of yoga that you could try. The simplest type to incorporate is gentle or relaxation yoga. This will focus on slow, gentle postures while incorporating breathing techniques, and occasionally a short meditation.

QIGONG – This is a practice that incorporates postures with breathing. The word Qi (pronounced chee) means 'life force' and it is through these postures that your life force is reinvigorated.

TAI CHI – This is actually a style of martial art where you are using your own internal energy to fuel movements in a rhythmic pattern.

Along with the above suggestions, you may also be interested in a leisurely walk. Walking, at whatever pace you can manage, is an excellent way to bring movement to your joints and increase your heart rate. Try walking in nature for a meditative effect.

There is no right or wrong way to incorporate movement into your life. Anything you add will help you to feel better. If all you can manage is 10 minutes at a time, then that is the right amount for you. Eventually, you'll be able to manage moving a few minutes longer. Progress!

# TRANSFORMATION IS BEGINNING

# 'WHY?' ISN'T AS IMPORTANT AS 'HOW?'

*"It is through gratitude for the present moment that the spiritual dimension of life opens up."—Eckhart Tolle*

After the shock of a diagnosis begins to dissipate, questions that often come afterward are 'Why did I get this? Or What did I do wrong? Or How did this happen?' This way of thinking keeps you in a state of constant stress and worry, which is unhealthy for you. Stress and worry will imprint in your body, creating physical symptoms, which will compromise your immune system.

## KATE'S STORY

*Kate was someone I met shortly after she was diagnosed. She described herself as a typical worrier, but with a cancer diagnosis the worry scale jumped through the roof. While she went through treatments, her only focus was why this had happened to her. Like what happens with most people, her foundation was shaken when she heard "You have cancer". Kate told me that that feeling never left her. Her mission became to find out why she got cancer and she turned into some sort of super sleuth along the way. To Kate, this entire situation would make sense if only she knew why. If only.*

*Kate grew up in a small, remote town and moved to a larger city to go to school. After graduating from university, Kate remained living in the city where she went to school, which was approximately a three hour drive from her immediate family. It wasn't always easy for them to travel to her and Kate really felt the distance as she went through her treatments and appointments.*

*However, Kate had developed a wonderful circle of friends, through work and social groups, some of them feeling like family to her. As any close friends would be, they were there for her during her time of need. They offered Kate their services. They brought her food and supplies. They checked in by phone and email. They took turns taking her to her chemo treatments and appointments. After each treatment, one of them stayed with her so that she would not be alone overnight. There was a lot of love being directed toward Kate.*

*You would not have guessed it however, by listening to Kate. Her attitude was still negative and worrying. Almost every conversation she had with someone was focused on why she became ill, with no focus on how she could become well. After a few conversations together, I finally asked her what it was that was driving this need and desire to understand why she developed cancer.*

*Her answer was this "If I can find out how I got it, maybe I won't get it again."*

*Wow!*

Kate is living in the future, while she lives in the past. She is so focused on why she got cancer so that she does not get it again, that she is forgetting how to move through it and get well. In addition to not focusing on how to help herself in this moment, she is missing seeing all of the love and healing that surrounded her at that time. Whatever opportunities and possibilities she could have gained to learn and grow from this experience were lost.

"*Are you there God? It's me Margaret. We're moving today. I'm so scared God. I've never lived anywhere but here. Suppose I hate my new school? Suppose everybody there hates me? Suppose they don't wash their hands after they use the bathroom? Suppose I get some terrible bacterial infection? Please help me, God. Thank you.*"—Excerpt from Judy Bloom, Are You There God? It's Me, Margaret.

Margaret turned out okay. So did Kate.

# You Don't Own 'Your' Cancer

*"Healing means getting over the pain, not marketing it."—Carolyn Myss*

People with cancer sometimes use interesting language when they reference what they have. You often hear phrases like "my lymphoma" or "my breast cancer" or "my tumour". Pause for a moment and think about that. Mine. The word 'my' is used to reference something that belongs to you; for example, 'my car'. When you own something, you are responsible for everything about it.

I would like to take the example of a car a little further. Let's say you decide you need a car so you select one that you like and then purchase it. Once you own the car, you are now responsible for oil changes, buying fuel to keep it going, cleaning it, changing tires and all of the other maintenance surrounding the ongoing life of the car. You might even give it a 'pet' name. You may even assign a gender, as in "careful, you'll scratch her".

People who have cancer can adopt a similar thought process. They think of cancer in terms of ownership, by categorizing it as 'mine'. When they say something like 'my tumour', does it belong to them and are they responsible for it? On the one hand, yes, it is in their body, so there is a degree of 'taking care' that needs to take place. However, it does not belong to them. It is not necessary to own it and make it theirs. By taking ownership of the cancer, it could extend the feeling that they are somehow responsible if it progresses.

If placing ownership on the cancer is how you refer to it, changing your perspective of owning the cancer in your body is a good place to start. Perhaps you could consider it an annoying guest that stays a little too long at a party. You take care of their needs while they are at your home, but you do not own how they behave.

By changing your perspective and the language you use, you begin to disassociate yourself from the cancer. Once you feel separate from it, you no longer feel responsible for it. This does not mean that you will not take care of yourself or your body and ignore treatments. It means that you no longer feel the burden that having it is your responsibility, or as an extension, your fault. Soon your attitude around taking care of it begins to change. It becomes something in your body that needs treatment to help it on its way, and not something you own that you need to tend to, care for and nurture.

## STELLA'S STORY

*Stella was 38 years old when she was diagnosed with breast cancer. She had been married for 4 years and had a young daughter. For the last ten years she worked for a bank in the mortgage department. She had gained many close friendships over the years with co-workers and clients.*

*When she was diagnosed with cancer, she was devastated. For the last two years, she and her husband were trying to get pregnant with their second child. The story of infertility was on the top of top Stella's mind and she received a lot of attention and support from the people around her. Now, with a diagnosis of cancer, her story shifted as she spoke of 'her' breast cancer.*

*When I first met Stella, I noticed that she often referred to the cancer as 'my cancer'. In every conversation where cancer was discussed, the reference was always about 'her' cancer. I noticed how Stella became protective of the tumour. It was a part of her; she owned it and it became her story. When she spoke about any issue or obstacle in her life, 'her' cancer was factored in the story. 'Her' cancer got in the way of feeling peaceful, of repairing a relationship, of her ability to maintain some of her usual tasks.*

*I suggested to Stella that she might want to join a support group, to have additional resources for herself. During one of her group sessions another woman, Julie, who recently discovered that she used to use the similar terminology, asked her why she said 'my cancer' all of the time. Stella said that because it's in her body, it is her responsibility. Julie shared her own story and that she realized that as soon as she made the connection to stop owning the cancer in her body, it became easier for her to let go and move on. A light bulb just turned on for Stella!*

Stella's story is quite common. When you are diagnosed with cancer, it can become your story and you may adopt a feeling of owning it. A simple shift in perspective lifts the burden of ownership and you can focus on taking care of the rest of you. You don't have to own it for healing to take place.

# FEELING HELPFUL, NOT HELPLESS

Changing a few letters changes a lot. There is a stigma that goes along with having cancer that a person is somehow rendered helpless. Meaning that they are unable to help themselves. That may be somewhat accurate in certain cases, however very often that is not always true. Certainly someone may need a little extra help if they have had surgery or feel weak after a chemo treatment. But for most people they have taken care of themselves for all of their lives, and are still qualified and capable.

When you are diagnosed with and in treatment for cancer and your energy is depleted, and people around you treat you as though you can no longer think for yourself, you may start believing them. You may begin to think 'no, I can't get my own glass of water' or 'no, I can't pick up my mail'. Perhaps you start to rely on the advice of others. Perhaps you do need someone to tell you to do the simplest of tasks; like when to shower, have a cup of tea or watch the news. A bit of an exaggeration, I know. Does this ring true for you?

The shift to feeling helpful is an empowering one when you are not feeling well. Once you become aware that you are considering yourself as 'helpless' you can easily shift that thought process to becoming 'helpful'. It is natural to feel good when you are helping others and doing things for yourself. You may not have full control of everything in your life, for example scheduling medical treatments, however you are definitely in control of your thoughts. Begin to start evaluating the areas of your life where you have control and then you can begin to initiate the 'helpful' you.

SOMETHING TO TRY...

Here are a few simple suggestions that will help encourage the 'helpful' you. Sometimes even the smallest thing can help you to feel the most empowered you have felt in a long time.

*Clear the table after a meal.*

*Reorganize a closet.*

*Drop off a bag of food to a local food bank.*

*Make a batch of muffins and give them to someone who has been a big help to you.*

# AFFIRMATIONS. SAY THEM OUT LOUD!

An affirmation is a phrase you state loudly to affirm what you believe or what you want to believe. This process can feel incredibly healing. There is something that happens when you say something out loud that makes us take notice and listen. Repeating it silently in your mind does not have the same effect.

There are studies that show how the language you use directly affects your body and surroundings. Looking at the work by Dr. Masaru Emoto, for example, shows how this could be true. Dr. Emoto was a researcher and alternative healer from Japan. He was fascinated by words, positive and negative, and how the energy of the words affected people. In one of his more popular studies, he used positive and negative words to create the formation of crystals.

For this experiment, he placed pieces of paper with positive and negative words on containers of water; each container had one piece of paper with one word. He then froze the containers. When the frozen water crystals were studied under a microscope, the water that had positive words written on them formed beautiful crystals. However when negative words were used the crystals did not form or if they did, they were not attractive. He also conducted a similar experiment by playing classical music and using prayer, with similar results. The study is subjective in that beauty is in the eye of the beholder.

Believe it? Many people do. But even if you are skeptical, try to consider how language or even using affirmations could be helpful in your healing process. In the book *Words Can Change Your Brain* (Newberg and Waldman), it states, "a single word has the power to influence the expression of genes that regulate physical and emotional stress". They suggest that we are hardwired to respond to certain words negatively or positively. By using positive words such as love, kindness or peace, our genes are affected and as a result the part of our brain that has to do with cognitive functioning is influenced.

The book also states, "By holding a positive and optimistic [word] in your mind, you stimulate frontal lobe activity. This area includes specific language centers that connect directly to the motor cortex responsible for moving you into action. And as our research has shown, the longer you concentrate on positive words, the more you begin to affect other areas of the brain. Functions in the parietal lobe start to change, which changes your perception of yourself and the people you interact with. A positive view of yourself will bias you toward seeing the good in others, whereas a negative self-image will include you toward suspicion and doubt. Over time the structure of your thalamus will also change in response to your conscious words, thoughts, and feelings, and we believe that the thalamic changes affect the way in which you perceive reality."

The idea that using one word can alter your body chemistry is an interesting concept when considering how it can influence cancer. One of the things I did after being diagnosed was to love the tumour in my body. Every day I told it "I love you", often more than once a day. I thanked it for appearing and teaching me whatever lessons I needed to move forward in my life. I intuitively felt that giving it love would help it to go away. Why would I love it? Not because I wanted the cancer to stay, but because I felt that if I accepted it for what it was, it would do what it needed to do and then move on.

The idea of affirmations is so mainstream now that it is not difficult to find a book or blog on this subject. One of the more popular authors in our time is Louise Hay. She wrote many books; however one of her more popular books is called *You Can Heal Your Life*. This book is an easy read and can help the reader to understand the idea of how what we believe creates our reality.

The suggestion to believe what you say to yourself is not a new concept. Your subconscious mind will believe your thoughts and images, whether they are real or not. If you are constantly in a state of worry, your mind registers these thoughts and your body reacts to them. However, if you use language that is loving, calm and true, then your body will react to that instead.

In an earlier section, Tuning In To Thoughts, being aware of the thoughts that are in your consciousness was discussed. This is an important and necessary step. In order to understand how your thoughts are affecting you, you first need to identify them.

If you have tried the exercise suggested where you set an alarm, tune in and then monitor your thoughts at the precise moment that it sounds, then you are learning to understand your thoughts and the messages you tell yourself.

*"Affirm the person you would like to become. Affirmations are simply a title for the things we say to ourselves about ourselves. Rather than thinking about who you have always been, start telling yourself who you are today in the present moment. As an example: "I am confident, powerful and decisive"—John Demartini*

## SOMETHING TO TRY... STATING AFFIRMATIONS!

You can choose a specific time of day, for example first thing in the morning, or you can state them whenever you feel you need them, whether they are daily or not. There is no right or wrong way. The key is to begin.

Here are a few affirmations from Belleruth Naparstek, a noted guided meditation expert.

I know that the more I can acknowledge and accept what I truly feel without criticism or blame, the more I assist my body's natural tendency to be well.

More and more, I consider the possibility that my body is teaching me something useful – that this cancer has been challenging me to learn and change and grow.

I thank my body for teaching me to love myself, express myself, stick up for myself and accept myself.

I know that when I can forgive myself and others for errors of the past, I allow my body to heal.

I invite assistance from my friends and loved ones, past, present and future to lend me their support and strength. I see myself surrounded by their loving caring and I can feel it all over my body like a warm wave.

I look inside my body and see vigilant, loyal, white blood cells, fierce and determined, scouting for cancer cells, surrounding them, penetrating them and destroying them with their powerful toxins. I can see this happening and I can feel this happening.

I look inside my body and I see the rebuilding of new cells, perfect, vital, healthy, aligned with the original blueprint. I can see this happening. I can feel this happening.

When I eat, I instruct my body to make use of what it needs and to reject whatever is unhealthy to me. I sense my body following these instructions.

When I go to sleep, I instruct my body to continue its healing at an even higher intensity than in my waking state and I sense my body following these instructions.

I tell this cancer these things, "Thank you for teaching me to stop and listen. Thank you for reminding me of what is truly important. YOU CAN GO NOW."

I know that I have things to do, gifts to give, purposes to accomplish; I require a healthy working body for this.

More and more, I know that I am held in the hands of God and I am perfectly, utterly safe.

A few simpler statements to try can be these:

I love myself.

I am well.

My immune system is healthy and strong.

I am a loving being and am worthy to receive God's love.

Every cell in my body is healthy, strong and energizing.

I am at peace.

I am joyful.

When you use affirmations, there is no wrong way to do it. It is all right because it is true for you. Use statements that feel true for yourself and your healing. It is important to include affirmations that resonate for you, even if you are not accustomed to using that language. What is important is that you believe that to be true. That you are worthy. If so, then state it. If you do not believe it, state it anyway. Because you are!

# HO'OPONOPONO

Within days of being diagnosed, someone told me about the Ho'oponopono prayer. I was vaguely familiar with it, but had not spent time researching or reading about it. At the time, I was willing to think 'outside of the box' and be open to anything that could help me so I started to consider what it was and how it could help me. I had not considered this as a method of healing an illness, but I do recognize that in clearing emotional stress, your body's chemistry begins to change. When I began using it, I soon discovered how energy shifted and changes happened for me.

Ho'oponopono surrounds the concept of reconciling, forgiving and loving persons and situations from one's past. The work became more popular when the book *Zero Limits* by Joe Vitale was published. There are workshops available and you can research them on www.hooponopono.org.

In ancient Hawaiian culture, it was believed that a person's past mistakes causes illness; that everything that becomes a problem began with a thought and the memories attached to these thoughts. It is these memories that are carried through generations and create problems- illness, arguments, etc. In the Hawaiian dictionary, Ho'oponopono is described as "family conferences in which relationships were set right through prayer, discussion, confession, repentance, and mutual restitution and forgiveness". The idea is that a senior member of the family facilitates a conversation whereby everyone is acknowledging, repenting and asking for forgiveness. Often they would look to an outsider, a 'healing priest', for assistance.

"If we can accept that we are the sum total of all past thoughts, emotions, words, deeds and actions and that our present lives and choices are colored or shaded by this memory bank of the past, then we begin to see how a process of correcting or setting aright can change our lives, our families and our society."—Morrnah Nalamaku Simeona, Ho'oponopono Master Teacher

It consists of four simple statements that are designed to clean your past, in order to bring love to your present. By intending, that is setting an intention of love and reconciliation with a person or situation, it sets in motion the process of healing.

## THE STATEMENTS

I LOVE YOU
is to direct love toward yourself

I'M SORRY
is to apologize to a person or situation for any wrong that may have happened, currently or ancestrally

PLEASE FORGIVE ME
is to ask for forgiveness from the person or about the situation

THANK YOU
is to thank yourself, the other person, the universe

What if healing could be this simple?

*I Love You*
*I'm Sorry*
*Please Forgive Me*
*Thank You*

## Linda's Story

*I put it to work. Shortly after I was diagnosed and in the process of arranging appointments with various doctors and such, I needed to connect with my family doctor in order to set paperwork in motion. In the back of my mind, I recall the doctor saying something about a 'rush' case so time was sensitive and therefore I was anxious. At the time, calling my doctor's office was nerve-wracking on a regular day. His nurse was very protective of him and his time. Good for him. Bad for me. Before calling, I put the Ho'oponopono to the test.*

*I imagined the nurse, sitting at her desk, being busy. I said the four statements, visualizing her, and then visualizing me phoning the office. After five minutes had passed, I made the call. It went smoothly, without any anxiety.*

*Was it the Ho'oponopono? I'm not sure, but I feel that it was. I felt calmer so it somehow changed the energy around the situation. Perhaps it was only me that had changed. It may be that I was able to reconcile something in myself that made calling the office challenging in the past. I can't say with certainty, but I believe it to be true. I had faith that this process worked.*

*I felt that if I could feel a sense of peace over a phone call, maybe I could feel and send peace to the tumour. I took it a step further and started repeating these four statements to the cancer in my body. Holding my hands over the tumour, I repeated:*

*I Love You*
*I'm Sorry*
*Please Forgive Me*
*Thank You*

*I can't tell you with any certainty that it changed the size of the tumour or the outcome, but it did change me. I felt a sense of peace and calmness surrounding me that I welcomed with open arms.*

Is this doing cancer right? Yes it is because it felt right for me. In that moment, it felt right. I had faith that it was making a difference for me. And in that faith, wherever the journey took me, I knew that I would be okay.

# HAVING A SPIRITUAL CONNECTION

*"Healing requires a willingness to make changes in both your physical and your spiritual way of life."*—Caroline Myss

# BE GRATEFUL IN EVERY MOMENT

Having gratitude for yourself and others has a positive effect on your body and mind. However, this can probably feel like one of the more difficult things to do when you have cancer. How do you muster up a feeling of being grateful when you are going through treatments, sometimes feeling pain and everything else that goes along with it? If you can give it a try, rather than feeling pain you may feel stronger, more alert and focused and have more joy.

Studies conducted at the University of California in Berkeley show that writing a gratitude journal will have a positive physical effect; for example increasing your immune system and lowering blood pressure. Participants in the study also noted feeling more joy and other positive emotions including having compassion for themselves and toward others.

Begin by simply stating each day "I am grateful for this moment and every moment that follows." When you are grateful in each moment life feels easier, people are tolerable and a glitch that would have bothered you in the past does not feel as bothersome.

When you are filled with gratitude there is little room for anger, envy or stress. As annoying circumstances emerge you will feel better able to cope because you have a foundation of gratitude. In moments when you are feeling your absolute lowest, stating that you have gratitude in that moment will not only change how you are feeling, but can also change your perspective about the situation.

## Something to Try...

Sit in a quiet space where you will not be distracted. Bring into your awareness a situation or person that has triggered a negative feeling or response. Either in your mind or out loud, state that you are grateful for the situation or person. Use some of these statements to get started.

*"I am grateful for this moment."*

*"I am grateful for my life."*

*"I am grateful for the people around me."*

*"I am grateful for each breath."*

*"I am grateful for each moment and every moment that follows."*

# FORGIVENESS IS ACCEPTANCE

> *"Forgiveness is the most powerful thing that you can do for your physiology and your spirituality. Yet, it remains one of the least attractive things to us, largely because our egos rule so unequivocally. To forgive is somehow associated with saying that it is all right, that we accept the evil deed. But this is not forgiveness. Forgiveness means that you fill yourself with love and you radiate that love outward and refuse to hang onto the venom or hatred that was engendered by the behaviors that caused the wounds."—Wayne Dyer*

Forgiveness is a big piece of your spiritual growth and will help you to move forward in your healing. Practising forgiveness enables you to overcome your situation by accepting that it happened, forgiving the person or event and moving on, which helps you to become stronger.

By allowing yourself to forgive, it is you who receives the gift. You benefit because you have let go of feelings of anger and hatred. These negative feelings, when held in for a long period of time, create stress in your body. By releasing these feelings you begin to feel better and to heal.

No doubt, one of the most difficult people to forgive is you. Think of some of the self-talk that happens in your mind. How often do you think or say something unkind about yourself? "I don't look good...I'm not smart...I'll never learn this", may be some of messages that you are telling yourself. More importantly, this internal monologue is occurring constantly and often goes unnoticed.

Where these messages come from is not important. What is important is the ability to release those thoughts so that you can begin forgiving yourself. The phrase 'just let it go' is one that you hear quite often. Usually it is said as a response when someone is unable to stop thinking or talking about a situation. Sometimes it can be that simple: just let it go. Other times, you need to do a little more to 'let go'.

## Something to try...

Think of a situation or person that you feel some type of negative emotion toward, be it anger, resentment or shame. State loudly, "I forgive (whatever or whomever) for (situation)". Repeat the statement. Notice how your body feels.

## Something to try...

During a meditation imagine yourself to be in a safe place and feel very comfortable. This could be a familiar place that you know of or a different place that you imagine. After spending a short time in this safe place, bring into your awareness a situation that occurred in the past that has been difficult to forgive. Let go of the attachment you have around the circumstances and begin to foster forgiveness for the person or situation. You may even want to have a brief chat with the person to try to understand their side of the story. If you notice a feeling of discomfort at any time, remember that you are in your safe place where conversations are calm and reflective.

Once you have finished your meditation, notice how you feel.

# Practice Compassion

After receiving a cancer diagnosis, people who do not consider themselves to be spiritual generally begin a spiritual journey. There is a small part in everyone that wants to know what life is all about and they are working toward 'nirvana' – that state of freedom from suffering. In Buddhism, nirvana is the final stage to transcendence where a person no longer suffers and has cleared any karmic debt. In order to reach nirvana you must complete the Eightfold Noble Path. This is step-based process of how to live your life in such a way that will help you to reach a state of peacefulness and love.

I have always considered it to be a good reminder on how I would like to live my life – see things as they are, have good intentions toward others, be kind with my words, to make a difference in the world in a positive way and finally, with meditation, to be accepting and at peace. Is this just something for Buddhists? Not at all. Imagine if all of humanity lived this way. The world would look a lot different than it does.

While Buddhism is one belief on how to live your life, there are many others. Certainly living a spiritual life is not only for people who belong to an organized religion. If you were to look at all religions you would find that their main goal is quite similar: to live a compassionate life where you are treating other people with love and kindness, in the way you would wish to be treated. It is the Golden Rule – Do not do unto others what you would not want them to do to you.

This idea of the Golden Rule is part of every religion. Karen Armstrong is an author and researcher of religions. She writes about the commonality held in all religions and is considered an expert in this field. She founded the Charter for Compassion in 2009.

One of my favourite quotes of Karen Armstrong about compassion states, "Compassion is aptly summed up in the Golden Rule, which asks us to look into our own hearts, discover what gives us pain, and then refuse, under any circumstance whatsoever, to inflict that pain on anybody else. Compassion can be defined, therefore, as an attitude of principled, consistent altruism."

I often wonder how my life would be different if the world was filled with compassion? Taking that thought further, how would the world be different if everyone had compassion toward each other, including their enemies or people whom they resent?

Compassion needs to begin within you. It is not enough to be compassionate only to other people, animals or groups. If you cannot foster compassion for yourself it will be even more difficult to extend that compassion to others. For if you do not recognize it, how can you extend it? Therefore, when you begin a process of forgiveness of self and accept yourself fully, you can then extend compassion to others.

The process of beginning to have compassion for yourself can feel daunting especially if it isn't something you have easily practised in your past. You may have experienced situations where someone has hurt you, where you have hurt others or moments of regret. This can trigger emotions in you from anger, sadness, and guilt to shame. When you hold on to these feelings, in your body and your mind, it creates physical symptoms leading to stress. This is where the disconnection from your spiritual self occurs.

To reconnect with yourself, you could simply begin a practice of meditation and use the time to focus solely on you. It is a beautiful gift to treat yourself as you would a good friend and to be completely self-aware. In each moment, accept and love yourself wholly and completely. Practising compassion toward yourself is the ultimate acceptance of who you are as a spiritual being.

## Time for Reflection

If you like, you can reflect upon the following questions and either meditate on or write about them in a journal.

1. Recall a time where a good friend or family member felt badly about himself or herself. How did you respond to them? What did you say to help them feel better?

2. Think of how you spoke to your friend in the previous question and then think of a time when you felt badly about yourself. Did you treat yourself in the same manner as your friend?

3. Recall a time in your life that you would do over if you had the opportunity. What would you do differently?

# AFTER ALL, I'M CONNECTED

Before I put pen to paper to begin writing this book I knew that I wanted to end here, with an emphasis on spirituality. For me, this section was the most important because it was a big part of my overall cancer experience. Also in the discussions I have had with many cancer patients, that it is in spirituality where they find the truest form of themselves. It is important to relate that regardless of how you approach cancer and regard the previous chapters in this book, that the key to doing cancer 'right' will find its foundation here—with the spiritual connection.

The statement above says a lot—after all, I'm connected. It says that I knew it was enough, would feed me throughout, would enable me to feel calm and was what I knew to be true. That the connection I had would help me to serve both myself, and then others. There is a comfort that comes with feeling connected to someone or something; somewhere where we find strength, peace and acceptance.

What is your connection? It could feel like God, Divine Being, Almighty, Lord or Yahweh. Your connection could also feel like a presence, with no association to a being of any kind. A source where you gain strength, find peace and comfort. The name is irrelevant, it is the feeling you have and what you receive from this connection that is most important.

When a person is diagnosed with cancer, many questions are flung to the forefront of their mind: What's it all about? What is my purpose? Where will I end up? Have I earned my place? And where is that place? There are many ways to discuss spirituality and the effect is has on a cancer diagnosis.

These questions are followed by many more, like what to do, how to do to it, who to see, where to go, how to live, what to eat, which medications are best. However, overshadowing all of it—every question, meeting, appointment, treatment, interaction—is this; that you are connected to something greater and that something greater is helping you guide your wellness. Once you know this (know meaning to understand it and feel how it relates to your core and beliefs), then everything seems to make sense.

And yes, having cancer can make sense. Sense in that there is a purpose to having cancer, if only to help you understand how cancer now fits into your life and the purpose your life serves you. Moving beyond that, understanding how your life serves other people in your life and society.

When I was diagnosed I referred to the cancer as a gift. It felt natural and right to say those words for I fully believed it to be true. I knew in that moment of diagnosis that having cancer was going to help me. I was going to learn what my purpose was, how I was able to handle a crisis, teach me humility, learn what my body could handle and understand emotional pain. This can sound a bit scary, but many of us know that it is through the difficult moments that we become strong and learn our biggest lessons.

I also knew that I was going to need someone else to lean on. It is beyond helpful to have a friend, spouse or family member that is there for you. It was a wonderful help to me having my husband's support and friends and family nearby that cared, called and visited. But I needed something else in addition to the people that I knew. I needed strength that went beyond the people around me. For me, I found that strength in my connection.

The idea that spirituality is considered a process of personal transformation resonates for many people, for it is in having cancer that you are transformed. It is in the process of having this illness, in all of its variations, that we learn, grow, understand, gain faith, change and therefore transform.

> *"You have brains in your head. You have feet in your shoes. You can steer yourself any direction you choose. You're on your own. And you know what you know. And YOU are the one who'll decide where to go..."*—Dr. Seuss

When I was diagnosed, I had an established relationship with god and I understood my place in the universe. I didn't question why this happened or what the purpose of my life was. That brilliant proclamation by Dr. Seuss so fittingly related to me. I understood that I was steering my wellness and the manner in which I was going to have this illness. I also understood that I was the one who would choose the thoughts I would have and maintain the relationships I valued as I continued to honour my spiritual path.

What I have discovered in my conversations with many cancer patients is that everyone is in the process of finding a way to live that is true for them. People with cancer want to incorporate changes and implement ways to cope that will help them while they are going through the illness and beyond. Many situations in life can be a catalyst for change and having cancer is one of those situations.

This conscious awareness is a gift I received from having cancer. I can choose my thoughts, my words and my actions based on being true to my authentic self. Something else that I have come to understand is that everyone who is diagnosed, whether they get well or not, is working toward the same goal: to find a way to live that is congruent with their authentic selves.

You may not have an established spiritual practice, and that is okay. This experience of having cancer is unlike anything you will know. The gift in all of this is the ability to explore what feels true for you. Whether it is partaking in a religious practice or simply knowing that you are part of a greater universe; it is in the exploration that our greatest lessons are learned.

## Jay's Story

*You could consider Jay to be a 'non-follower' of anything. He hadn't considered himself to be religious or spiritual. Growing up, he went to services with his family, but stopped going as soon as he left his childhood home. Like so many people, he thought something was there, but never invested any time trying figuring it out or to understand how the concept of god fit into his life as an adult. His life was busy and although having a spiritual practice was important, it wasn't important enough to begin doing something about it.*

*After Jay was diagnosed with lung cancer at the age of 37, he reconsidered the importance of spirituality in his life. Jay began a journey of discovery that stays with him today. When he was told he had cancer, the one thought that kept swirling around in his mind was that he 'just wanted to get through this so that everything could go back to normal'. Jay didn't realize at the time that his normal was no longer the same. He slowly began to realize that life automatically changes when you have cancer and rather than wishing everything*

110

*would go back to the way it was, it's important to embrace what is to come.*

*He always felt that he would be okay and physically heal. He knew it in his heart and never felt as though he needed to be afraid of the word 'cancer' or the physical effect it was having on his body. If you asked him today how he was so certain, he would say that there was a 'knowing' inside that he felt. He would even go as far as to say that it was a voice, guiding him.*

*To reconnect with his spirituality, Jay felt it was important to feel a connection to something. It was a feeling that was missing for him all of these years and it wasn't until having cancer that he wanted to find it again.*

*Jay began by researching. He read many books, researched information, listened to current spiritual speakers and he found a series of steps that helped him. He began his day with meditation, in order to tune into his thoughts and tune out what he didn't need in the moment. Jay then incorporated prayer into his daily practice. He asked for healing for himself, others and the planet. He also began learning how to let go of resentments and practise forgiveness. In his interactions with people he made an effort to treat every person with kindness and discovered that the kindness extended from him and outward toward others.*

*Jay's spiritual journey changed. He became focused on his purpose, his true self and his desire to live in a way that felt peaceful and loving. As a result his relationships changed for the better, he felt peaceful and he was able to move through cancer with confidence and ease.*

*Jay is in remission now. He told me that one thing he attributes to his healing was, ironically, being diagnosed with cancer; because had he not been diagnosed, he would not have rediscovered what was missing—his connection.*

## TIME FOR REFLECTION

If you like, you can reflect upon the following statements and questions and either meditate on or write about them in a journal.

1. If you have considered any self-transformation practices in the past, what were they and how do you feel about them now?

2. How would you like to develop your spiritual practice further?

3. Think of a spiritual teacher, past or present, read some of their work and reflect on what meaning this has for you.

# ACKNOWLEDGEMENTS

I would like to thank my friends who helped me along the way while writing this book. For those of you who listened, read, line-edited and provided feedback, I thank you. The book would not have been written without your help. Truly.

To my husband, Joseph: you were with me during cancer and nursed me throughout, you continuously encourage me to find my life's path and support me in every way. I am grateful and I thank you.

# ABOUT THE AUTHOR

Linda Morinello lives in Niagara Falls, Canada with her husband. She is an Integrative Nutrition Health Coach, speaker and facilitator. She has worked with numerous clients and runs her practice from her home, conducting sessions in person, phone and Skype. She is also a Program Leader for Wellspring Niagara, facilitating various programs and workshops for cancer patients and their caregivers.

Linda spends much of her time reading, researching and attending workshops and conferences in order to further her knowledge and to help her clients. When she isn't working, you can find her in her kitchen creating healthy dishes and sharing recipes with clients and friends. Linda says, "Cooking is my meditation. When I'm creating, I feel fulfilled and re-charged."

She is currently working on her next book. For more information about Linda, please visit www.good4me.ca.

*Notes*

*Notes*

*Notes*

CPSIA information can be obtained at www.ICGtesting.com
Printed in the USA
LVOW08s0349020915

452286LV00005B/139/P